Evaluation of the Hospital Board and the Chief Executive Officer

Richard P. Moses

AHA®

American Hospital Publishing, Inc.,
a wholly owned subsidiary of the
American Hospital Association

The views expressed in this book are those of Richard P. Moses.

Library of Congress Cataloging-in-Publishing Data

Moses, Richard P.
Evaluation of the hospital board and the chief executive officer.

Bibliography: p.
"Catalog no. 196123"—T.p. verso.
1. Hospitals—Trustees—Self-rating of. 2. Hospital administrators—Rating of. I. Title. [DNLM: 1. Governing Board—organization & administration. 2. Health Facility Administrators—standards. 3. Personnel Management—standards. WX 150 M9104e]
RA971.M636 1986 362.1'1'068 86-17319
ISBN 0-939450-98-4

Catalog no. 196123

Printed in the U.S.A.
2.5M-10/86-0162
2.5M-4/87-0180
2.5M-11/88-0227

Beryl Dwight, Editor
Peggy DuMais, Book Production Coordinator
Brian Schenk, Editorial and Acquisitions Manager, Books
Dorothy Saxner, Vice-President, Books

No one ever knows us quite as well as we know ourselves.

—*Sigmund Freud*

Contents

Foreword

Introduction

Part 1. Self-Evaluation of the Hospital Governing Board

Prologue 2
Organization of the Board 3
Charter and Bylaws 3
Selecting a Chairman of the Board 5
Size and Composition of the Board 9
Committee Structure and Function 12
Trustee Selection and Development 15
Functional Areas of the Board 19
Mission Statement 19
Quality of Care 22
Financial Responsibility 25
Evaluating the Chief Executive Officer 28
Community Relations 31
Image in the Community 31
Media Relations 34
Market Share and Acceptance 36
Board-Medical Staff-Administration Relations 38
Joint Conference Committee 39
Medical Staff Involvement in the Board 41
Board Involvement in the Medical Staff 44
Joint Retreat/Seminar Meetings 46
Long-Range/Strategic Planning 49
Board Involvement in the Planning Process 50
Monitoring and Evaluation 52

Part 2. Evaluation of the Chief Executive Officer

Prologue 56
The CEO Evaluation Process 57
Determining the Procedure 57
Subjective and Objective Evaluation 61
The CEO's Role in Planning 64
Mission Statement 64
Long-Range/Strategic Plan 66
Specific Goals and Objectives 68
Day-to-Day Functions of the CEO 70
Leadership Ability 70
Employee Relations 73
Board-Management Relations 76
Role in the Community 78
Medical Staff-Management Relations 80
Contracts for the CEO 82
Incentive Compensation for Executive Management 85

Foreword

Richard Moses has undertaken a challenging task—describing a process for the self-evaluation of the hospital board and for the board's evaluation of its chief executive officer. The challenge has become acute today because of the many changes wrought in the management and governance of hospitals through the impact of political, social, and economic influences on the provision and delivery of health care services to the American public.

Hospital boards and their management teams have been bombarded during the past two decades with a myriad of changes, known in boardrooms by such acronyms and initialisms as TEFRA, PPS, DRG, PSRO, PRO, HMO, PPO, and IPA. The roles and responsibilities of the hospital board and its CEO have had to change radically as a result. In the past, the formulation of hospital policy dealt with the growth and expansion of the hospital. Not so today—policies formulated now speak to the future of hospitals and their survival in the face of increasing competition from every corner of the health care field.

Consequently, a hospital board and its chief executive officer can ill afford to take their performance for granted, and evaluation of their performance becomes essential. The purpose, of course, is not just to discover how well they are doing, but also to give them an opportunity to know how to improve.

The challenge undertaken by the author has been well met. Any board member or chief executive officer, experienced or otherwise, will find helpful insights and practical suggestions throughout this book, which is commended to their attention. Appropriately used, the book will aid the development of qualities so essential to effective board and management operations—qualities such as a forward-looking attitude, a clear definition of the responsibilities of all parties, a firm commitment to the cause served by the hospital, and a confident expectation of development and progress in response to the external forces affecting hospitals today.

Use it well!

George Wm. Graham, M.D.
Consultant
Chicago, Illinois

Introduction

Meaningful evaluation of performance has been a long sought-after but elusive goal of business. Most of the businesses we are familiar with tend to measure effectiveness of performance by equating it with economic profitability. Indeed, daily newspapers, trade journals, and special business publications routinely report earnings, profits, dividends, and, for publicly held companies, daily stock quotations.

Corporate directorships, which health care facilities are being urged to emulate, are usually judged solely on the balance sheet performance at the end of the year. Yet, in today's world of corporate failure, we must ask ourselves if there are other vital criteria for assessing board performance. This book is an attempt to address that question as it relates to hospitals.

The book is divided into two parts. Part 1 deals with areas of board responsibility that should be included in an effective self-evaluation by a hospital governing body. Part 2 deals in more detail with one such responsibility—evaluation of the chief executive officer.

Following each section or chapter is a checklist that board members can use for evaluation of their hospital, their chief executive officer, themselves, or their governing body as a unit. These checklists may be copied for internal or not-for-profit use without written permission from the publisher, as long as the credit line appears on each reproduced page.

Many individuals encouraged me in the writing of this book and have made me acutely aware of the responsibilities of trusteeship. I will refrain from mentioning any of them for fear of overlooking someone. They know in their hearts who they are, and for both their friendship and advice, I am forever grateful.

Richard P. Moses

Part 1
Self-Evaluation of the Hospital Governing Board

The governing body evaluates its own performance.

—Joint Commission on Accreditation of Hospitals
Accreditation Manual for Hospitals, 1986, Section 4.1.19

Prologue

John Addison was rather frustrated. About a year ago he had been flattered at being asked by the chairman of the board and the chief executive officer to serve on the governing board of Carlson Memorial Hospital. He felt sure that his past record of civic service was a prime reason for this invitation, and he took pride in what he had done for his community.

Now, after a number of meetings of the hospital board, he was not sure that this was exactly his cup of tea. It seemed to him that meetings were largely devoted to a lot of minor matters that really should be handled by the CEO. Of late, there had appeared to be an increasing amount of factionalism in the board; motions had been both carried and defeated by narrow margins, indicating a lack of unanimity among the board members. He knew there were committee assignments made at the beginning of the year, but the committee he was on had never met, and he had not heard a report from other committees except for one or two some months ago.

John's feeling of frustration was shared by several other members of the board. Accordingly, they gave their full attention when a consultant assisting with the annual retreat planning asked, "Has the board ever undertaken an evaluation of its own performance?"

Organization of the Board

How the board is organized and how it handles its own development and growth are vital functions that enable the board to carry out its total responsibility effectively.

Charter and Bylaws

The board is governed by an approved set of bylaws derived from its charter. The charter and the bylaws are the very soul and substance of the hospital. Their contents should be clear, complete, up-to-date, and easy to read and understand. Too many times these documents are judged on their volume and not on their content.

All board members need to have a good knowledge of the contents of these two documents. This does not mean that they should be able to quote chapter and verse, but they should know where to find particular topics in them. Usually the rules of the governing board provide that all members of the board be furnished a current copy of the charter and the bylaws when they begin their term of office.

These documents of governance need to be reviewed on a regular basis; usually this is done by a special committee that is charged with that responsibility. Because the health care field continues to change dramatically, changes in the charter and the bylaws of the hospital may also be required. Just as the mission statement of the hospital should be regularly reviewed, so should the documents that govern the hospital's performance.

Checklist—Charter and Bylaws

Instructions: *Rate the following statements in relation to your hospital and governing board. Rank each answer from* **5** *(strongly agree) to* **1** *(strongly disagree) or answer* **yes** *or* **no**.

1. All members of the board are furnished a copy of the charter and the bylaws when they begin their term of office.	____Yes ____No
2. The charter and bylaws have been reviewed or revised within the past five years.	____Yes ____No
3. I believe I have a good knowledge of the charter and the bylaws.	5 4 3 2 1
4. I believe that the board abides by the charter and the bylaws.	5 4 3 2 1

Selecting a Chairman of the Board

Next to the chief executive officer, no other person is more important to the governing body than its chairman, who is the representative of the hospital at all times and greatly affects the public's perception of it. Therefore, the selection of this person is of utmost importance to the board and should be done carefully and with a great amount of consideration. Too many times we see the chairman's position merely rotated among the board members, either by seniority or by previous position held (as, for example, when the secretary's position is considered a stepping stone to the chairmanship). Instead, this important position should be filled on the basis of merit and ability.

Because it is desirable to have different leaders in this position, the term of the chairman should definitely be a limited one. Accordingly, the bylaws of the governing board should provide a carefully thought-out process for both the selection and length of service of the chairman.

The chairman has two basic areas of responsibility: the hospital and the community. At the hospital the chairman is the recognized leader of the governing body. More than any other person, he or she determines the pace at which the board moves. In addition to all the responsibilities connected with the conduct of meetings, the chairman usually is responsible for all committee appointments, serves as liaison with the medical staff either on a formal or informal basis, and is available to the CEO for consultation on a regular basis. The chairman may also be called upon to participate in various negotiations that take place within the hospital in any number of settings.

In the community the chairman wears the mantle of the hospital at all times. Here also he or she may be involved with various government bodies in negotiations that affect the hospital. The chairman is expected by the businesses and industries in the community to be receptive to their concerns about health care. This expectation is also true of various civic organizations, clubs, and other entities in the hospital's community.

The chairman of the board should be a respected, successful leader in the community, a good public speaker, and a person who "presents" well before groups. He or she therefore needs a thorough background and knowledge of all facets of the health care system, the environment, and the community needs for health care.

As noted, it is highly likely that the chairman is going to be involved in some sort of negotiations with local government bodies, outside agencies, members of the medical staff, and members of the administrative team of the hospital. In this position as negotiator, the chairman needs to be a person who possesses unusual traits and talents and, above all, who is respected for ability and acumen.

Finally, the chairman should be an innovative and forward-thinking person, willing to take risks and to lead the board into venturing beyond the accepted practices of the past.

Checklist—Selecting a Chairman of the Board

Instructions: *Rate the following statements in relation to your hospital and governing board. Rank each answer from* **5** *(strongly agree) to* **1** *(strongly disagree) or answer* **yes** *or* **no**.

1. There is an orderly, prescribed method for the election of a chairman.	5 4 3 2 1
2. The chairman is selected on the basis of merit and ability for the position.	5 4 3 2 1
3. The term of the chairman is included in the bylaws and specifies a set number of years.	____Yes ____No

Checklist—Self-Evaluation by the Chairman of the Board

Instructions: *Rate the following statements in relation to your performance. Rank each answer from* **5** *(strongly agree) to* **1** *(strongly disagree).*

1. I start meetings promptly at the appointed time.	5	4	3	2	1
2. I use parliamentary procedure as necessary and the rules of order prescribed in the bylaws.	5	4	3	2	1
3. I am familiar with all the items on the agenda.	5	4	3	2	1
4. I am fair to all board members and do not show favorites.	5	4	3	2	1
5. I appoint necessary committees promptly, with the approval of the board.	5	4	3	2	1
6. I am available to the chief executive officer on a regular basis.	5	4	3	2	1
7. I am a leader in board education and development and support board member attendance at seminars, retreats, and so forth.	5	4	3	2	1

Size and Composition of the Board

No formula exists that dictates what size a hospital board should be or just what composition will be in the best interest of the hospital. Surveys conducted by various organizations show a wide range in number of members. The average board size, according to a 1985 American Hospital Association survey, was 14. Sometimes outside factors affect the size of a hospital board; often, law or other considerations remove this decision from the board itself.

Generally speaking, a board should be large enough to ensure community representation and to carry out its necessary functions effectively. If the board is rather small with numerous working committees, members may think they are overworked and that the hospital is demanding too much of their time. But if the board is so large that it is cumbersome to carry out its duties, members may become frustrated, and their interest may wane as they try to accomplish the functions of governance. The size of the board should be such that members feel comfortable with it.

In considering the board's representation of the community, the geographic distribution of board members should be taken into account. It is not desirable for all of the board members to come from one particular area of the community, as this situation may foster a sense of isolation in other parts of the hospital's service area or make it appear that the hospital is being run by a clique or special-interest group.

It is difficult for a hospital to have its fingers on the pulse of the community if its board membership is confined to one segment of the populace. I am not suggesting that the community should be parceled off into wards or precincts with specific representation from those areas, as is often the case in city or county government. Nevertheless, a board should regularly look at the residence address as well as the business address of its members to make sure that the geographic distribution doesn't become too narrow.

Boards need a variety of business perspectives in their decision-making process. Because of their varied backgrounds, board members will bring to the decision-making process important and different views that are helpful in arriving at the best approach to a particular matter. Board members, however, should not be expected to render professional service by reason of their occupation. For example, although there might be a certified public accountant (CPA) on the board, that individual should not be asked to render some service in the area of the hospital's accounting practice. The same holds true of attorneys, engineers, and so forth.

The governing board also needs to look regularly at the age of its members. Otherwise, it is easy for a board to find that the average age of its members has passed beyond a desirable figure. Although no magic number exists that a board should strive for, the board should continually seek a good age distribution among its members. Industry has long recognized the need for bringing on younger people as the age of its board membership creeps upward. We in health care very much need the infusion of ideas and the desire for change that young people can contribute.

Some boards set a mandatory retirement age for their members, whereas others allow extended service. I believe that a mandatory retirement age should be agreed on by the board members and should be strictly observed because it is important to make room for others who are younger to come on the board. Retired board members can still serve through advisory committees or emeritus status.

Another means of limiting the length of board service is by setting a maximum number of consecutive years or terms that a board member may serve. This period is often established in the bylaws as nine years or three three-year terms. Although bylaws may allow for a certain number of consecutive terms, more than one term should never be automatic or be considered a right.

Checklist—Size and Composition of the Board

Instructions: *Rate the following statements in relation to your hospital and governing board. Rank each statement from* **5** *(strongly agree) to* **1** *(strongly disagree) or answer* **yes** *or* **no**.

1. The board is large enough to carry out its necessary functions effectively.	5	4	3	2	1
2. The composition of the board is representative of the community.	5	4	3	2	1
3. There is fairly good geographic distribution of board member residences.	5	4	3	2	1
4. A variety of business backgrounds and perspectives are represented on the board.	5	4	3	2	1
5. The age distribution of board members is good.	5	4	3	2	1
6. A mandatory retirement age from the board has been set and is strictly observed.	5	4	3	2	1
7. The maximum number of consecutive years or terms that a member may serve has been set and is strictly observed.	5	4	3	2	1

8. In my opinion, the board is:

too small	____Yes	____No
too large	____Yes	____No
the right size	____Yes	____No

Committee Structure and Function

If ever there was a functional organization dedicated to the principle of committee operation, the hospital is it! There is usually a committee for just about anything that has to be carried out in the institution. So it is with most governing boards. An important factor in accomplishing goals and objectives through committee activity is the structuring of the committee and its charge. Some board committees appear to be formed at the drop of a hat, given very little direction as to purpose, and, most important, not given a specific time frame in which to accomplish their work. Also, many boards have standing committees that seldom meet and that have little purpose in existing but look important on the organization chart.

A hospital board needs appropriate committees to carry out specific charges so that the board can function at its best level of performance. Obviously, the committee needs are different for the board of a 1,000-bed teaching hospital and the board of a 150-bed hospital. However, in determining how many committees each one needs, the same principle should apply: a board should have only those committees that are absolutely necessary for it to receive the information needed to make sound judgments on pertinent issues. Remember, committees seldom have the authority to make decisions for the governing body but are usually expected to bring recommendations to the board so that the board can make an intelligent decision after carefully reviewing all the information at hand.

The size of a committee may necessarily vary with the type of work that is expected of it. For example, a committee that is supposed to get a community reaction to a new service the hospital is considering might be many times larger than a committee that regularly reviews the property insurance values of the hospital. However, both committees need to know exactly what is expected of them and the time frame in which their work is to be completed.

Some standing committees have a responsibility to make regular reports to the board, whereas ad hoc committees are created for a specific purpose and often function for a limited time. An ad hoc committee should be disbanded when it has completed its work.

Boards sometimes think that all committees should be composed solely of board members, but there is a wealth of talent within the hospital itself, as well as in the community, that can assist in committee work. Often, a committee may need the expertise of the medical profession, or it simply may be in the interest of all concerned to have medical staff participation on a certain committee. If there is an advisory group or committee, these members are also a good source of committee membership outside of regular board and medical staff.

In summary, committees should be structured as to size, membership expertise, and a time frame consistent with the task they have to accomplish. A committee that functions by doing the necessary research, considering all the alternative actions that can be taken, and then making a clear and concise report to the governing body can be of invaluable assistance in the board's decision-making process.

Checklist—Committee Structure and Function

Instructions: *Rate the following statements in accordance with the facts of your hospital governing board. Rank each answer from* **5** *(strongly agree) to* **1** *(strongly disagree).*

1. The structure and purpose of committees are set forth in writing, with all members of the board notified.	5	4	3	2	1
2. Ad hoc committees are created for a specific purpose, have a time frame, and are disbanded when the purpose has been achieved.	5	4	3	2	1
3. Regular reports from committees are given to the board or to the appropriate body.	5	4	3	2	1
4. Minutes of all committee meetings are kept in an appropriate manner.	5	4	3	2	1
5. Where possible, board members are allowed to indicate a preference for the particular committee on which they would like to serve.	5	4	3	2	1
6. Where appropriate, individuals other than board members are asked to serve on committees of the board.	5	4	3	2	1
7. Where appropriate, members of the medical staff are asked to serve on committees of the board.	5	4	3	2	1
8. Individuals designated as committee chairmen have usually demonstrated leadership ability and have a basic knowledge of the activity their committee is to pursue.	5	4	3	2	1
9. All standing committees are regularly reviewed to make sure that they are necessary for the governance function.	5	4	3	2	1

Trustee Selection and Development

It is essential that the governing body have a well-thought-out process for the selection and orientation of new board members. A board that is self-perpetuating, that is, that selects its members when a vacancy occurs, should first examine the make-up of the current board as to age of members, their geographic distribution in the community, and how well they represent the business and socioeconomic elements in the community.

Those boards that do not have the prerogative of selecting new members to fill a board vacancy should try to have an input to those who *do* make the selection. If the decision rests with a political body like a county council, the governing body should convey its views to the council as to the needed "talent" on the board. If left solely to its own choosing, a political body will often make a political appointment, and this can be to the detriment of the composition of the governing board. In some states, hospitals are considered public service districts, and, as such, their board members are elected by the public. In such instances, the public must be well-informed about the hospital and its needs.

How does one find good board members in the community? Persons who have a demonstrated sense of civic service should be sought out. Those who have been active in any type of volunteer work, such as the Red Cross, scouting, United Way, church work, or Chamber of Commerce are people who have indicated a willingness to serve their community in a volunteer manner. Boards should have persons who are recognized as community leaders and who are on the forefront of activities for the betterment of the area in which they live. Boards should strive to identify persons who have high moral and ethical standards, who are well-respected by their peers, and who are successful in their chosen field of endeavor.

An advisory group or committee, if present, is excellent as a source of prospective board members and as a means of developing and recognizing leadership abilities.

As individuals, board members should possess:

- Willingness to become thoroughly knowledgeable about the health care field
- Commitment to serve the community through the hospital
- Willingness to make decisions after full consideration of all the options

- Ability to compromise when there is an honest disagreement over action to be taken
- Willingness to work with others as a team
- Ability to represent the views of the hospital to the community and the views of the community to the hospital
- Willingness to devote the necessary time to the business of hospital governance

The manner in which a person is asked to serve on the board of a hospital is important. It should be done in a dignified and businesslike setting that is conducive to conveying the responsibility of what the prospective board member is being asked to do. Often persons are approached in a social or relaxed setting, such as a party, that is not compatible with the position they are being asked to accept.

If the board has developed a position or job description for its members, it may be a good idea to let prospective members see in writing just what will be expected of them. Prospective members should also understand that there is a written policy on conflict of interest for board members. In our eagerness to have someone accept the position we have offered, we may tend to minimize or to paint a glowing picture of the work to be performed. This can cause major problems later on when the new member of the board realizes rather abruptly just what hospital governance is all about!

It is incumbent upon the board to make sure that a well-planned orientation process has been implemented that will provide the new trustee with a beginning education in the health care field and the responsibilities and authority of the governing board. By starting out with a sound orientation program, a board will find that in the months ahead it can expect a level of performance that will make the new member an asset to the board and not a liability.

Perhaps no subject has been more publicized in governance circles than the need for trustee development and continuing education. Usually lacking in the rhetoric about this subject is any kind of consensus as to just what the ingredients are for a planned, systematic development program that continues throughout the year. Too many boards believe that having some kind of program once a year will satisfy the needs of the board.

Many boards have found that using seminars, conferences, or the like is the best method of providing board development. Some boards will set aside some time at each meeting or at a planned time in the year for this purpose. Other boards will go a long distance away from their community and spend two or three days in a retreat setting for discussions on present status, future directions, or strategic planning. Whatever suits the board best should be the overriding factor in deciding how to achieve board development.

Whether a trustee development activity is conducted by in-house staff or an outside agency, the board should participate in the planning process. An outside agency should be used only as facilitator; trustees more than anyone else know the subjects in which they think they are deficient and just what it is in this changing world of health care that they want and need to know more about.

Many boards involve members of the hospital medical staff or physicians from the community in this development process in order to establish better understanding and a more cooperative attitude between the two groups. Such activities should be done in an orderly, planned manner, with stated goals and objectives to be accomplished.

One of the true measures of trustee development is the ability of the board to meaningfully evaluate its own performance. This process is an excellent indicator of board deficiencies and also provides a method for curing those deficiencies.

To ensure appropriate procedures for selection and development of members, the governing body should establish:

- A selection process for members that ensures, insofar as possible, well-qualified, dedicated individuals to serve on the governing body
- A written position description that fully informs individual board members of their duties and responsibilities
- An orientation program that enables new members to fully understand their responsibilities in serving on the governing body
- A continuing education program that assists board members in keeping abreast of the health care system
- A goal of achieving diversity of membership as to age, geographic distribution, socioeconomic factors, and business interests, without selecting members as representatives of special-interest groups

Checklist—Trustee Selection and Development

Instructions: *Rate the following statements in relation to your hospital and governing board. Rank each answer from* **5** *(strongly agree) to* **1** *(strongly disagree) or answer* **yes** *or* **no**.

1. The board (for those boards that are responsible for selecting their members) has a well-defined, written policy on how the selection process is carried out.	5	4	3	2	1
2. The selection process for board membership is done in a manner that ensures broad community representation and divergence of interest.	5	4	3	2	1
3. A written position description for new trustees sets forth the responsibilities of the individual members and of the board.	____Yes		____No		
4. There is a written policy on conflict of interest to which all members of the board subscribe.	5	4	3	2	1
5. The orientation program gives new members the opportunity to become familiar with the hospital and the governance process.	5	4	3	2	1
6. The board plans, adopts, and sets forth a program for trustee development at least annually.	5	4	3	2	1
7. The budget of the hospital includes the necessary funds for trustee development.	5	4	3	2	1
8. The board includes members of the medical staff and administration in education programs that will be of benefit to those groups.	5	4	3	2	1

Functional Areas of the Board

Certain areas of board activity are on the agenda of board meetings on a regular basis. They do not necessarily occupy more of the board's time in discussion but are subjects that boards find they must deal with on a meeting-by-meeting basis.

Mission Statement

The mission statement of the hospital sets forth the purpose of the hospital, its goals and objectives, and the way in which it plans to meet the health care needs of the community it serves. Usually the mission statement defines the hospital's service area and states the level of health care it is attempting to provide.

The mission statement needs to be clearly and precisely written, easy to read and understand, and such that it can be widely disseminated to the publics served by the hospital. Its intent will be defeated unless it is written to indicate just what the institution intends to do in rendering health care to the community it serves.

To write a mission statement that is totally out of touch with reality or so broad in its wording that it is meaningless to those who read it is truly an exercise in futility. Furthermore, any person reading such an ill-prepared document will usually be frustrated in trying to understand just what the hospital intends to accomplish. Indeed, instead of finding support among the populace, a hospital may find it has created an adversarial situation. The mission statement should be a living, viable, changing document that at any time can be used as a reference point to make sure that the hospital is on target regarding the delivery of health care to the community it serves.

Both the medical staff and the administration should have input in the preparation of the mission statement; in addition, some governing boards like to have participation from community representatives. Usually the mission statement of the hospital is reviewed annually or, at the most, biannually. This review may be done by a board committee or by the entire board.

Many hospitals publicize their stated goals and objectives to the community by means of the mission statement. The publicized statement therefore becomes a way of facilitating better understanding between the hospital and the community.

Checklist—Mission Statement

Instructions: *Rate the following statements in relation to your hospital and governing board. Rank each answer from* ***5*** *(strongly agree) to* ***1*** *(strongly disagree) or answer* ***yes*** *or* ***no.***

1. I have read and am familiar with the mission statement of the hospital.	5 4 3 2 1
2. The mission statement clearly sets forth the goals and objectives of the hospital.	5 4 3 2 1
3. The board seeks and is receptive to input regarding the content of the mission statement.	5 4 3 2 1
4. The mission statement is reviewed by the board or a board committee at least every two years.	_____Yes _____No
5. The mission statement is well publicized to the community.	5 4 3 2 1

Quality of Care

The governing body has no greater responsibility than that of striving to ensure that the highest possible quality of care is being rendered in the hospital that it governs. Although this authority is usually delegated to or at least shared with the organized medical staff, the board is not relieved of what is termed the ultimate responsibility in this area of health care. In case after case, the courts have held that the legal responsibility for the overall quality of care rendered in the institution rests with the governing body.

This area of board activity requires a dedication and perseverance often misunderstood by many board members. After all, the great majority of boards are composed of laypersons who are untrained in the medical profession but who have to render judgments in this field. As difficult as it may seem, striving to ensure a high quality of care is a board function of the utmost importance and one that should be given a considerable amount of time. No longer can boards afford merely to rubber-stamp matters of quality of care that come before them from the medical staff or some hospital committee.

Most hospitals have a formalized quality assurance (QA) program that is designed to ensure that the high quality of care that the board desires is being carried out. The board should receive regular reports regarding this program, and a means of liaison between the board and the quality assurance committee should be established. Obviously, the organized medical staff plays an important role in this area, and the board needs to be assured that all participants in the quality assurance program are carrying out their responsibilities as required by the charge to the QA committee.

Risk management is an increasingly important area of trustee concern in quality-of-care issues. Board members should be aware of the hospital's insurance coverage for malpractice liability, its history of liability claims and losses, and any additional claims as they occur.

The credentialing process by which physicians are admitted or reappointed to the medical staff is a vital area of quality of care. Here again, much of this responsibility is shared with the medical staff, but the board has the final responsibility of giving approval to the individual seeking admission or reappointment to the hospital's medical staff.

In the past, and still lingering in today's governance, some boards have rubber-stamped their approval of medical staff recommendations. With the growing supply of physician and non-physician practitioners, hospitals are going to be under increasing pressure to admit a greater number of individuals to their medical staff, and the credentialing process is going to be an increasingly important part of the governing board's activity. In fact, the Joint Commission on Accreditation of Hospitals, in its accreditation process, spends a major amount of its time in surveying this area of hospital activity.

The board's granting of specific privileges once an individual has been admitted to the medical staff is another complex area of quality of care. It is often an even more sensitive area than that of the original admission to the medical staff. For example, doctors may feel that they need to expand or change their practice pattern and will seek permission to do this through a request for additional privileges. To enable the board to carry out its responsibility, a mechanism is necessary to ensure that such physicians possess the necessary clinical competency to perform in the area in which they seek the additional privileges.

The hospital governing board needs to be assured that the process of determining clinical competency at all levels is functioning well and that it is not subverted or short-circuited by some means. In addition, the board should be familiar with the procedures established in the medical staff bylaws for disciplinary action against a member of the medical staff and should be notified of any such action taken.

Checklist—Quality of Care

Instructions: *Rate the following statements in relation to your hospital and governing board. Rank each answer from* **5** *(strongly agree) to* **1** *(strongly disagree) or answer* **yes** *or* **no**.

1. There is a well-functioning quality assurance program that makes regular reports to the board.	5 4 3 2 1
2. A means of liaison has been established between the board and the quality assurance committee.	____Yes ____No
3. The board is immediately notified of any hospital-related malpractice claim.	5 4 3 2 1
4. The board or a board committee takes an active and well-defined part in the credentialing process.	5 4 3 2 1
5. Applications for admission or reappointment to the medical staff are reviewed by the board or a board committee and approved by the full board.	5 4 3 2 1
6. A change in or granting of privileges for practice is done with board approval.	5 4 3 2 1
7. The board is notified of any disciplinary action taken against a member of the medical staff.	5 4 3 2 1
8. The board is familiar with the written procedure to ensure due process in a disciplinary action involving a member of the medical staff.	5 4 3 2 1
9. Members of the board regularly attend some phase of the survey process of the Joint Commission on Accreditation of Hospitals.	5 4 3 2 1

Financial Responsibility

The financial affairs of the hospital have long been the darling of hospital boards. One of the longer-held tenets of governance and one that has been constantly emphasized to governing boards is their responsibility for the assets of the institution and its financial viability. Many new members coming on the board have the perception that they are expected to bring to the board a certain financial expertise that will help the hospital in better utilizing its resources and in containing costs. In the early annals of the history of health care, it is said that private hospitals that operated at a deficit during the fiscal year merely divided up this deficit amongst the trustees, who were expected to "ante up" their share of this figure! Perhaps this long-discarded practice is what makes board members think that considerable time and expertise will be required of them to ensure the financial soundness of the hospital.

The complexity of health care accounting and all of the attending financial practices often overwhelm the average board member. It is a language and practice that is so foreign to most trustees that after a while they may throw up their hands in surrender and merely accept as correct all of the many financial statements that are presented to them. However, diligent and conscientious board members will find that the financial statements of hospitals, although different from anything with which they may be familiar, can be understood and can be a source from which they can make sound judgments in determining the future direction and allocation of resources for the hospital.

The board should receive monthly financial statements that clearly indicate the performance of the hospital against stated and budgeted goals and objectives. These goals and objectives are part of the budgeting process that usually takes place at a time appropriate to the hospital's fiscal year. The board has to give final approval to the budget, and the review process is usually done by the finance committee or a special committee. If the budget is unrealistic in a certain area of operation, making an adequate assessment of the financial performance of this area will be difficult. Also, as "bricks and mortar" monies become increasingly scarcer, it is incumbent upon boards to be more diligent in their financial planning.

Hospitals usually break their budgets down into at least two categories, operational and capital expenditures. Often, it is not easy to separate the two completely because they interact with each other, and a budget item may have a direct effect in both areas. However, it does help the board to see these two budget categories and to understand what the goals and objectives of each are.

The board is expected to make a final determination on the margin of operations, or bottom line, that it expects from the hospital's yearly income and expense. As the fiscal year progresses, it is important for the governing body to be kept well-informed of all areas of financial operation. There should be no surprises in this vital area of activity that could cause a major upheaval in the institution's operations. It may also be necessary for the board to amend the budget as the year progresses and unforeseen changes take place. These changes could be of a positive nature but still such that they would require a restructuring of some financial matters.

The board is charged with the responsibility of selecting the financial institutions with which it wishes to do business. This may include investment counseling firms, bonding institutions, or banking institutions that the hospital deals with on a day-to-day basis. The arrangements with these institutions should be reviewed on a regular basis and the services being rendered compared with other services that are available. Often the finance committee or a similar committee is charged with this responsibility by the board. It should be noted that this is an area of activity that may present a conflict of interest for bank board members or bank employees who serve on the hospital's board of trustees.

The board also has a similar responsibility in the selection of the firm that does the annual audit of the hospital's fiscal affairs. The audit should be made available to all members of the board, and it should be reviewed diligently. To receive direct input from the auditors, many boards will ask the auditing firm to meet with them or a committee of the board.

Checklist—Financial Responsibility

Instructions: *Rate the following statements in relation to your hospital and governing board. Rank each answer from* **5** *(strongly agree) to* **1** *(strongly disagree) or answer* **yes** *or* **no.**

1.	The board or a board committee has a major role in determining the budget of the hospital.	5 4 3 2 1
2.	The board or a board committee sees detailed monthly financial statements of operation.	5 4 3 2 1
3.	The board determines the bottom line of operation for the hospital.	5 4 3 2 1
4.	The chief financial officer or a representative of the accounting department makes regular reports to the board on the overall financial well-being of the hospital.	5 4 3 2 1
5.	The board is kept current as to accounts receivable, indigent care, and bad debts of the hospital.	5 4 3 2 1
6.	There is a separate budget for capital expenditures and operations.	_____Yes _____No
7.	An orderly process has been established for determining the financial institutions with which the hospital does business.	5 4 3 2 1
8.	The board votes on the firm selected to do the financial audit of the hospital.	_____Yes _____No
9.	The board or a board committee reviews the audit in detail.	5 4 3 2 1

Evaluating the Chief Executive Officer

I don't think I've ever met a chief executive officer who did not want to know what the board thought about his or her performance in the hospital. Yet often when the subject of evaluation is raised, an uncomfortable look appears on the CEO's face that usually means either the board has not done any kind of a performance evaluation or the job it *has* done has not been done well. Good CEO evaluation is of utmost importance if the board and administration are to work harmoniously and to have a complete agreement on just where the hospital is heading. Without this agreement, a board and administration may be at odds and may have different "agendas" regarding the hospital's future and its mission in serving the community. This section briefly describes some key aspects of board evaluation of the CEO. Part 2, Evaluation of the Chief Executive Officer, is a more detailed discussion of this important board function.

Like so many other tasks of the board, CEO evaluation should be done by a committee or some small body that represents the board. There probably is no reason to have more than three or four persons involved in the actual evaluation process; this number can vary in large hospitals or hospital systems. It is perfectly all right and proper for the full board to have discussion with and input to the committee that is going to do the evaluation; however, these comments and opinions should be conveyed to the CEO through the select committee. To call a CEO into a board meeting and have 10 or 15 people questioning his or her performance is counterproductive and will not result in a satisfactory evaluation of performance.

Most boards that are conducting CEO evaluation do it annually. There is nothing to prohibit its being an ongoing process, however, done quarterly or semiannually or with some other time frame that is agreeable to all concerned. It is important that it be done in a timely manner, when and where specified, and that the results be conveyed to all concerned. The evaluation process should be strictly confidential and so treated by the board and the CEO.

The methodology of evaluation as well as the criteria for evaluation must be agreeable to both parties. Remember that the CEO better than anyone else knows his or her performance and can greatly assist in this vital area of governance.

A certain amount of evaluation is subjective by nature, but much is objective; this objective evaluation provides the true measure of performance. The process means first sitting down with the CEO and agreeing on certain goals and objectives to be accomplished within a given time and then, at evaluation time, determining the degree of accomplishment achieved. The results of the evaluation are used as the basis for setting new or revised performance goals and objectives.

Some hospitals use incentives, usually related to compensation, as a means of rewarding exceptional performance. Here again, it is necessary for both parties to have a complete understanding of the level of performance required in order to secure these incentive rewards.

Checklist—Evaluating the Chief Executive Officer

Instructions: *Rate the following statements in relation to your hospital and governing board. Rank each answer from* ***5*** *(strongly agree) to* ***1*** *(strongly disagree).*

1.	The board follows a written policy in evaluating the performance of the chief executive officer.	5	4	3	2	1
2.	The CEO participates in setting any objectives on which the evaluation will be conducted.	5	4	3	2	1
3.	All members of the board are informed of the timing of the CEO evaluation and have an opportunity for input to it.	5	4	3	2	1
4.	The actual evaluation process is done by a small committee of not more than three or four members of the board.	5	4	3	2	1
5.	Whenever possible, objective criteria are used in evaluating the CEO's performance.	5	4	3	2	1
6.	The evaluation committee informs the CEO and the full board of the results of the evaluation.	5	4	3	2	1
7.	The results of the performance evaluation form the basis for new or revised performance goals and objectives.	5	4	3	2	1
8.	If incentives are offered, both the CEO and the board have a clear understanding of the criteria and procedure involved.	5	4	3	2	1

Community Relations

Acceptance in the community it serves is essential for a hospital. A health care facility may provide the highest quality of care in a handsome structure, but unless those in its service area have this perception, the facility will probably lack for utilization. It has been said that the buying public is fickle by nature, and this seems especially true of today's consumer of health care. A hospital cannot "hide its light under a basket" and expect the public to continue to use the facility simply because it is there. Today's rapid transportation usually offers an alternative to the sick or injured individual seeking health care, just as alternatives have been available for years for those having elective medical procedures or diagnostic testing.

The buzz word in the health care field today is *competition*, and therefore the entire matter of community and public relations takes on an even greater importance in the well-being of the hospital. Having decided that it wants a good image in the area it serves, a hospital must next decide just how to accomplish this. Although this section isn't meant to be a manual on public relations, it should provide governing board members with some insight into how good a job their hospital is doing in this important area.

Image in the Community

Some hospitals find out about their image in the community by conducting a survey. Such a survey can range from a sophisticated, in-depth poll, usually done by an outside firm, to a small sampling poll, done either in-house or with some minimal help from a support group. Some hospitals have used local teaching institutions or other sources of available community talent to assist them in a public relations project.

The following broad guidelines will help in conducting a survey:

- The governing body should play a major role in deciding how to determine the image of the hospital it governs. If a survey is decided on without the input of the board, the survey results may well be suspect when they are put before the board. Conversely, if the board has played a major role in this undertaking, board members are going to be quite interested in helping with the survey process and making sure that it accomplishes what it has set out to do.
- Whatever method a board may choose, it is of utmost importance that the information resulting from the survey be what the board was seeking. If the right questions aren't asked or the particular information that the board wanted is not obtained, then the opinion poll or survey is going to be of little value.
- A clear understanding and agreement among the board, administration, and, usually, the medical staff should be reached as to what any public relations poll should accomplish in gathering opinions from the public. And like so many things, it is best to have this in writing.

The results of any public relations survey should be used in determining major changes that may be contemplated within the hospital. Such results should not be the sole determining factor but should serve as a tool for the board in making decisions regarding immediate changes or the future direction of the institution.

Many hospitals use some sort of a patient evaluation form to sample, on a random basis, the opinions of patients after discharge from the hospital. This can be a simple one-page form or an elaborate and detailed questionnaire. It usually covers a wide range of subjects and is helpful in determining how patients perceive they were treated while in the hospital. It is intended to deal with the clinical as well as the operational aspect of their stay. Some forms ask for the patient's identification and others can be completed anonymously; there are advantages and disadvantages to each method. Some CEOs will share with the board or a board committee member the results of these surveys on a regular basis. This information helps board members gain a first-hand look at the way the public feels about their hospital.

Checklist—Image in the Community

Instructions: *Rate the following statements in relation to your hospital and governing board. Rank each answer from* **5** *(strongly agree) to* **1** *(strongly disagree) or answer* **yes** *or* **no**.

1. The hospital has a good image in the community.	5 4 3 2 1
2. The hospital has done a public relations survey.	5 4 3 2 1
3. The hospital uses a patient evaluation questionnaire on a random sample basis.	____Yes ____No
If *yes* to the above: This information is shared with the board.	____Yes ____No
4. The governing board is aware of and concerned about its image in the community.	5 4 3 2 1

Media Relations

It has often been said that a smart person or an organization does not do battle with those who buy ink by the gallon and paper by the ton! The same principle holds true for the air waves controlled by radio and television. Simply translated, this means that the hospital should always strive to have good relations with the news media by attempting to avoid adversarial situations.

Good media relations won't just happen; achieving them takes work. An important first step is trying to understand the mind-set of the media concerned. The bread and butter of the news media is news. They might be sympathetic to what a hospital is trying to accomplish, but if they don't see something as newsworthy, they're not going to be interested in using their valuable time and space in publicizing it. If there is something they consider newsworthy, however, it will doubtless receive attention in the media at their discretion, whether the hospital wants it publicized or not. The key is for the hospital to try to get the information it wants into the news and to try to keep what may be damaging to the institution from being publicized.

The news media expect complete honesty at all times. They may forgive a person once, but if they find that someone is rarely completely honest with them and tends to slant the information given them, they will become suspicious of that person as a source of news that is worthy of their consideration. Once the confidence of the news media has been lost, it is difficult to regain; it is far better to try to maintain a high degree of respect from them. When this has been accomplished, they are an invaluable ally; conversely, if they think they have been wronged, they can be a mortal enemy.

The health care industry is a complex business, and not all news media personnel may be familiar with it and all of its ramifications on the public. Often it is only necessary to educate media representatives on a health care issue in order for them to present it fairly to the public. Misunderstanding probably accounts for more bad coverage of a health-related matter then any other single cause. If the media are uninformed on a particular matter, they may easily mislead the public without intending to do so.

Checklist—Media Relations

Instructions: *Rate the following statements in relation to your hospital and governing board. Rank each answer from* **5** *(strongly agree) to* ***1*** *(strongly disagree) or answer* ***yes*** *or* ***no****.*

1. The hospital has designated someone who is responsible for public relations.	____Yes		____No		
2. The hospital enjoys good media relations in the community.	5	4	3	2	1
3. The hospital makes a conscientious effort to keep the media informed of major happenings at the institution.	5	4	3	2	1
4. When appropriate, the media are invited to meetings of the governing board.	5	4	3	2	1

Market Share and Acceptance

The past few years have seen a radical change in the way hospitals do business. Words such as *marketing, market share, advertising,* and *competition* were hardly known to the industry ten years ago. Today these concepts are of utmost importance to health care institutions, and public relations is closely intertwined with them. A hospital can survive only if it fulfills a need in the area it serves; the need has to come from the people, and the people have to acknowledge that the hospital is their choice for themselves, their families, and their employees. Without this acceptance, the prognosis for the survival of the hospital is not good. Therefore, the governing body needs to be aware at all times of the market share that its hospital is able to attract, and it should consider ways to improve that figure.

Statistics are available that show where patients in the area are going for their health care. Also, the patterns of physician referral should be studied to determine whether the hospital is getting its share of these referrals.

Several factors influence where patients go for their care today. Given a choice, patients may now pick one hospital over another; in the past, this decision was generally made by the physician, and the patient rarely took exception to it. In addition, a fierce competition is now evidencing itself among providers (such as health maintenance organizations, preferred provider organizations, individual practice associations, and businesses contracting with case management firms) that are determining where patients may go for hospitalization.

Checklist—Market Share and Acceptance

Instructions: *Rate the following statements in relation to your hospital and governing board. Rank each answer from* **5** *(strongly agree) to* **1** *(strongly disagree) or answer* **yes** *or* **no**.

1. The hospital is aware of its market share and its acceptance in the service area.	5	4	3	2	1
2. The board is aware of patient-origin data for the hospital.	5	4	3	2	1
3. Information on patient-origin data is shared with the medical staff.	5	4	3	2	1
4. The hospital is active in marketing its services in the area.	5	4	3	2	1
5. The hospital is well-informed regarding its local competition.	5	4	3	2	1
6. The governing board is aware of the competitiveness of the health care field.	5	4	3	2	1

Board-Medical Staff-Administration Relations

It has been said that there are no more complex business relationships than those that exist in today's health care institutions. Indeed, when we look at the forces at work in the hospital and consider their effect, it is a wonder that hospitals operate as efficiently as they do.

The medical staff is truly the life blood of the health care system; without physicians there would be no hospital. Then there is the administrative staff—highly educated and of a professional standing that is envied by many businesses. They represent the corporate head of the hospital and are charged with the day-to-day operations of this complex entity. Over these two bodies is the governing board, usually consisting of laypersons who are not professionally trained in their governance responsibility and who often have other business interests as well.

The courts have long established that the governing body has the ultimate responsibility for what happens in the hospital; the Joint Commission on Accreditation of Hospitals and other national health care organizations have long reflected this view. In order to carry out its responsibilities in the many facets of institutional governance, the board delegates to the medical staff and to the administration authority for certain matters in their particular areas of expertise. Although the board may delegate this authority, it cannot delegate the final responsibility, which rests solely with the governing body. Accordingly, it is not difficult to understand why the relationship of the board, medical staff, and administration to one another is of vital importance in the delivery of health care.

Joint Conference Committee

A mechanism needs to be established for the medical staff, the board, and the administration to meet on a regular basis to discuss matters of mutual interest. One of the more formal means of accomplishing this communication is a joint conference committee (JCC). A typical membership structure for such a committee might be the executive committees of the board and medical staff, with the chief executive office as one of the nonmedical members. There are many variations of committee structure, however, and it is just a matter of what works best for the groups involved. Meetings should be scheduled well in advance at a time and place that is convenient to all members.

Both the board and medical staff members of the JCC should have input to the agenda for meetings. A common practice is for the board chairman and the chief of staff to meet ahead of time to decide on the agenda. It is also desirable to allow other members of the JCC to submit items that they wish to have brought up at a JCC meeting. This practice does not mean that every item submitted will be put on the agenda, but it at least gives JCC members the right to submit ideas and to have them considered by those responsible for the agenda. Whatever the final agenda, it should be distributed to all those attending well in advance of an actual meeting.

Any action taken by the JCC should be reported at regular meetings of the board and medical staff. Normally, the JCC adopts recommendations that are taken back to the full medical staff and governing body for approval. If either of these bodies believes that decisions are being made by a small, close-knit group without their approval, there is a good possibility that the JCC will be thwarted in its efforts. Full support by members of the board and medical staff is essential for the success of the JCC.

Remember, the JCC should be a problem-solving body. Because the groups can best communicate with one another at this level, the committee should be viewed as a means of avoiding crisis situations or those issues that cause confrontation or adversarial relations. By defusing potential problems and approaching them in a positive manner, this committee can render an invaluable service in the maintenance of good relations among the board, medical staff, and administration.

Checklist—Joint Conference Committee

Instructions: *Rate the following statements in relation to your hospital and governing board. Rank each answer from* **5** *(strongly agree) to* **1** *(strongly disagree) or answer* **yes** *or* **no***.*

1.	There is a joint conference committee (JCC) composed of members of the board, medical staff, and administration.	____Yes ____No
	If *no*, omit questions 2 through 5.	
2.	The JCC meets on a regular basis.	____Yes ____No
3.	An agenda is provided well in advance of the meeting for those planning to attend.	____Yes ____No
4.	The JCC regularly informs the board and the medical staff of its meetings and its actions.	5 4 3 2 1
5.	The JCC is a problem-identifying and problem-solving committee.	5 4 3 2 1

Medical Staff Involvement in the Board

Although not as heated now as it once was, the debate still continues about members of the medical staff serving on the governing body of a hospital. A 1985 survey by the American Hospital Association shows that approximately 77 percent of responding hospitals have one or more physicians on their board. Perhaps the most traditional arrangement is to include the chief of staff as a member of the board and as a representative of the medical staff. If not a voting member, the chief of staff is usually extended the privilege of entering into any and all discussions.

In addition to the chief of staff, there should be some other physician membership on the board as well. Unlike the chief of staff, however, such physician members of the board are not representatives of the medical staff. This kind of physician membership on the hospital board should be much like any other membership on the board. Board members should be chosen for a variety of reasons, and these criteria should be the same in determining physician membership. A physician is not elected to the board to be a representative of other physicians any more than an accountant is elected to be a representative of other accountants. A physician brings to the board a certain desirable quality and an expertise in the health care field, much as other professionals bring with their background.

Some boards have used a numerical approach to set physician membership, and others have just left it open. Whatever the selection procedure, physician members of the board must fully understand why they have been chosen and what their responsibilities are. If this is not done, there is a fairly good chance that some conflict may arise because of a misunderstanding of the role of the physician board member.

Another method of involving the medical staff in the governing body is through membership on the various board committees. Medical staff members have much to offer, and it is just good common sense to call on this talent by having them participate in the committee activities of the board. Not only will they bring a special perspective to these committees, they will also be of invaluable assistance in trying to accomplish what the committees are charged to do.

Interacting through a committee assignment provides members of the board and medical staff with the opportunity to develop a good working relationship. Each group needs to understand the other, and this committee membership can be a big step in that direction.

Committee membership also can be a kind of screening process for prospective members of the governing body. This participation gives medical staff members an insight into just how the board functions, as well as indicating to the board just how interested the medical staff members are in governing board affairs.

Medical staff members of board committees achieve a direct input into the decision-making process that takes place in the board room; medical staff members of the board participate directly in this process. At both levels, this interaction and involvement can go a long way in developing harmonious relations between the board and the medical staff.

Checklist—Medical Staff Involvement in the Board

Instructions: *Rate the following statements in relation to your hospital and governing board. Rank each answer from* **5** *(strongly agree) to* **1** *(strongly disagree) or answer* **yes** *or* **no**.

1. There is good input from the medical staff in the decision-making process of the board.	5 4 3 2 1
2. Members of the medical staff serve on the board.	____Yes ____No
3. Members of the medical staff serve on committees of the board.	____Yes ____No

Board Involvement in the Medical Staff

The board has certain expectations of the medical staff by reason of the authority that the board delegates to the staff, such as in the area of quality assurance. By regular reports from the medical staff, the board wants assurance that the functions of the medical staff are being carried out properly. If the board merely rubber-stamps all the actions of the medical staff, it is shirking its responsibility in the governance of the hospital and may well find itself in difficulty later when and if some problem arises. Trusteeship neglect in the area of delegated responsibility to medical staff, specifically in credentialing, has resulted in some of the largest malpractice-related awards against hospitals.

In some hospitals, board members who are not physicians serve on committees of the medical staff. Although it is not as widespread as having physicians serve on the board, an argument can be made for this arrangement. Medical staff committees that meet without any input from the board are missing a vital ingredient in the decision-making process of the institution. This arrangement also keeps the board aware of the functioning of the various medical staff committees. Committees can often benefit from having an outside or lay opinion to consider when arriving at a solution to a problem. A further advantage of outside membership on medical staff committees is that it tends to make the so-called medical mystique a little better understood by the lay members of the board. Any structure that helps with this understanding will make for better relations and a more smoothly functioning hospital.

Checklist—Board Involvement in the Medical Staff

Instructions: *Rate the following statements in relation to your hospital and governing board. Rank each answer from* **5** *(strongly agree) to* **1** *(strongly disagree) or answer* **yes** *or* **no**.

1. Members of the board serve on or attend some meetings of the medical staff.	____Yes ____No
2. The board receives regular reports from the medical staff in areas such as quality assurance, in which authority has been delegated to the medical staff by the board.	5 4 3 2 1

Joint Retreat/Seminar Meetings

Perhaps the most popular and in some instances the most successful way of building good relations in a hospital is through a joint retreat or seminar meeting. This can be an elaborate affair lasting for two or three days or a simple one-day program. Although sometimes held in a resort-like setting, such a meeting can be held at the hospital itself or at some facility close by.

Several key points should be remembered, however, in planning for and carrying out this type of function. The meeting should be structured to appeal to the medical staff, the board, and the administration. Members from all three of these groups should be present, and each should feel that the time spent has been worthwhile. If the program is promoted to these three groups and if they know early on that their attendance is vital both for them and the hospital, their participation is fairly well assured. It is also an advantage to include a member from each of the three groups in the planning of the program. Often, the executive committees of the board and the medical staff meet with members of administrative staff to plan the topics to be covered and the mechanics of the meeting.

An added benefit from this type of planning will be that those involved will feel a kind of ownership of the program and will have a strong interest in making the function a success. Too many times, a program is planned for the board or the medical staff without consulting either of these bodies to see whether it is one of interest and current value to the members. It is not difficult to find out what is on the mind of trustees or physicians when planning a program. Just submitting a "market basket" of subjects for them to consider can be of great assistance in making sure that a program is on target. Even when a CEO has a definite idea about what the groups need to hear or know more about, it is wise to submit this plan to the two groups in advance for their reaction to it.

A retreat or seminar can also be a good way of giving detailed information on a subject that might be before the board or medical staff at a particular time. Such programs have been used to further the decision-making process in everything from a building program to corporate restructuring to joint ventures. Indeed, any kind of subject that is being considered for action at any time can be the focus of such a program.

Governing bodies sometimes think that once they have held a retreat weekend, nothing else needs to be done. Nothing could be further off target. For one thing, these types of meetings should be a continuing process, and there is nothing wrong with holding more than one a year. Also, these meetings lend themselves to follow-up meetings—not on the same scale as the original, but ones that are supportive of the action taken at a weekend meeting or a seminar. By setting the tone for future actions to be taken, these retreat meetings can well be the springboard for other action by the interested parties.

The social aspect of retreats is important and should receive considerable attention in the planning process. Most programs that are for more than one day allow some time for social or recreational activities. Many hospitals include the spouses of members in the program, providing an excellent opportunity for these different groups to get to know one another and to visit in a relaxed setting. This type of camaraderie can be of great benefit in the future when there are hard decisions to make in the hospital. As individuals become better acquainted in a setting that is less business-oriented, it is often easier to reach decisions in the business setting of a formal meeting.

Checklist—Joint Retreat/Seminar Meetings

Instructions: *Rate the following statements in relation to your hospital and governing board. Rank each answer from* **5** *(strongly agree) to* **1** *(strongly disagree) or answer* **yes** *or* **no**.

1.	The board has held a joint retreat or seminar within the past 12 months.	____Yes ____No
	If *no*, omit questions 2 through 6.	
2.	The retreats or seminars are held on a regular, scheduled basis.	5 4 3 2 1
3.	Members of the medical staff and administration attend board retreats or seminars.	____Yes ____No
4.	The planning for such programs is done with input from those who will attend.	5 4 3 2 1
5.	The program at the retreat or seminar is informative and of current interest to the groups attending.	5 4 3 2 1
6.	The retreat or seminar is an enjoyable occasion.	5 4 3 2 1

Long-Range/Strategic Planning

Probably more material has been written about, more meetings conducted in the name of, and more consultants hired in the cause of long-range or strategic planning than any other subject in the health care field. So important is this function that the Joint Commission on Accreditation of Hospitals lists providing for institutional planning as a standard for a hospital governing body. Hospital governing boards are constantly reminded of their obligation in this vital sphere of activity, but few really understand just what it is all about or just what they are supposed to do.

The cornerstone of any planning process is the mission statement, which should be referred to during the planning process to ensure that the hospital's mission and its plans are compatible. Of course, the mission statement is intended to be a changeable document and not something cast in concrete. Indeed, it *must* change as the mission of the hospital changes, and this of course is what planning is all about.

Based on the mission statement, the long-range plan should lay out the framework for the direction the hospital intends to go and should be like a road map in helping the hospital get where it wants to go for the next 5, 10, or 20 years. The planning process also requires the setting of goals and objectives—priorities must be established, funds budgeted, and time frames specified.

This chapter sets forth some minimum considerations for governing boards in carrying out their responsibilities in the planning process.

Board Involvement in the Planning Process

Hospital boards vary widely in their degree of involvement in the planning process. Many hospital boards simply leave this task to administration and then approve or disapprove the finished product that is submitted to them. Other hospitals hire a planning consultant to write the plan for them. Sophisticated, large hospitals usually have a full-time planner on their staff who is charged with providing the planning process necessary for the institution. Often there are combinations of these arrangements. There is nothing wrong with any of these methods of planning; some may work better for some boards and others for other boards. I personally like to see considerable input from the board members to the planning process.

The medical staff also plays a major role and should always be afforded a seat at the planning table. In almost every instance, medical staff support is going to be needed; the best way to ensure this support is to have members of the medical staff involved in the process as it develops. Remember also that the medical staff can be either an invaluable asset in the accomplishment of goals and objectives or a formidable adversary in blocking them.

If a board is to be truly responsive to the community, it must bring that responsiveness to the planning process. Only through understanding its community can a hospital be assured that its plan is on target for what it hopes to accomplish in the years ahead. A hospital that plans in a vacuum without any input from the community may find itself committed to an expensive undertaking that never really gets off the ground simply because there is no need for it. But a hospital that sets out through careful research and planning to meet a demonstrated need in the community will usually find itself successful in this endeavor.

Boards may decide to publicize their planning expectations to the community. Some hospitals may not want to publicize an undertaking until it is almost a certainty; nevertheless, a hospital may earn a certain amount of community support by sharing goals and objectives that are developed under the planning process. When those in the hospital's service area observe an orderly and constructive planning process taking place, they will tend to have more respect for the hospital and to be more supportive of its efforts.

Checklist—Board Involvement in the Planning Process

Instructions: *Rate the following statements in relation to your hospital and governing board. Rank each answer from* **5** *(strongly agree) to* **1** *(strongly disagree) or answer* **yes** *or* **no**.

1. The hospital has a structured planning process.	5	4	3	2	1
2. I am satisfied with the planning process and the manner in which it is done.	5	4	3	2	1
3. I believe that the degree of board involvement in the planning process is adequate.	5	4	3	2	1
4. The medical staff has input in the planning process.	5	4	3	2	1
5. The views and needs of the community are considered in the planning process.	5	4	3	2	1
6. The board uses the planning process in the setting of goals and objectives for its operation.	5	4	3	2	1
7. The results of the planning process are publicized in the community the hospital serves.	5	4	3	2	1

Monitoring and Evaluation

Monitoring both short- and long-range plans as they are put into effect is both necessary and desirable. If a board has set realistic goals to be accomplished in a set time, it can truly critique its performance under the planning process. For example, a hospital might have a goal of establishing a freestanding diagnostic center within a year. By regular reports and a monitoring process, the board can determine whether this project is being undertaken properly and is expected to be completed at the designated time and within budget. In case of an unforeseen incident that might cause a delay, the board can adjust the time frame and financing as necessary and still keep the project on track.

The board needs to monitor its long-range plan closely to make sure that it remains up-to-date and viable. Alterations and changes may occur, just as the needs of the community change, but by using the planning process and reviewing the plan regularly, a hospital can do its best to meet the needs of the people it serves.

Some governing bodies choose to have outside consultants come in to evaluate their planning process. This procedure usually ensures that the board will receive an unbiased and reliable opinion. If the consultants are fully qualified and if the board fully understands what the consultants are doing, this type of evaluation can be of considerable benefit to the board. Such outside consultants should be chosen with great care and should have a good "track record" in evaluation of planning to help ensure that the board is receiving sound advice in the critique of its planning process.

Checklist—Monitoring and Evaluation

Instructions: *Rate the following statements in relation to your hospital and governing board. Rank each answer from* **5** *(strongly agree) to* **1** *(strongly disagree) or answer* **yes** *or* **no***.*

1. The board adopts long-range as well as short-range goals under the planning process.	5 4 3 2 1
2. The board sets realistic time frames for carrying out its plans and whenever possible adheres to these time frames.	5 4 3 2 1
3. The long-range plan of the institution is reviewed on a regular basis.	5 4 3 2 1
4. The planning process is evaluated.	5 4 3 2 1
5. The governing body is informed of the evaluation of the planning process.	_____Yes _____No

Part 2

Evaluation of the Chief Executive Officer

Prologue

He had been the chief executive officer at Haygood Hospital for more than 22 years. A recognized leader in the community, he had served first as president of the Rotary Club and later as the district governor. Active in church work, he had also held leadership positions in the Boy Scouts on a regional and national basis. He was a fellow of the American College of Healthcare Executives and had served on the Blue Cross-Blue Shield board as well as the state health systems agency.

For some months, there had been rumors about feelings of dissatisfaction by some board members concerning his performance. Ever since the board had been restructured, over a year ago now, he had heard some of the talk that had been going around. However, the chairman of the board and others had assured him this was nothing more than idle gossip and not to be concerned about it.

The restructuring of the board had almost doubled its size, and no one felt quite the closeness and camaraderie that had existed prior to that action. As the months went by, it became evident that certain members of the board were less than pleased with the chief executive officer's performance. More and more it seemed that he was asked to excuse himself from meetings, usually near the end of regular board meetings. Sometimes there were special meetings of the board to which he was not invited.

One day the chairman summoned him and suggested that he consider early retirement. By then it was a foregone conclusion that he would either be fired or asked to resign; the latter action he took within two weeks' time.

Despite the increasing concern on both sides regarding the CEO's performance, the board of Haygood Hospital had never done an effective evaluation of its chief executive officer.

The CEO Evaluation Process

The key to any evaluation is its fairness. If either party is not completely satisfied with the process that is to be used, the evaluation is almost doomed from the start. Also, criteria that are going to be the basis for the evaluation must be agreed on. This, of course, requires input from the CEO as well as the board.

Determining the Procedure

The governing body needs to adopt a written policy that sets forth the methodology to be used in the evaluation of the CEO. Although minor changes may be necessary from year to year, the document should be permanent and should not change materially even though the board composition may change or different people may be involved in the evaluation.

Because many evaluation considerations carry over from year to year, the evaluation committee is one board committee that should have continuing membership in order to ensure the necessary continuity. Committee members should serve at least a three- or four-year period, with no more than one or two members who are new to the committee at any given time. The committee that is actually involved in the evaluation process should be rather small: usually no more than three to five members, depending on the complexity of the evaluation and the size of the board. In a committee of this size, it is absolutely necessary that all members actively participate in the committee function.

Although the committee will carry out the actual evaluation, this does not preclude input from the entire board itself. In fact, if board members are not allowed input into the evaluation, they may well feel that the evaluation has been performed in a slanted or incomplete manner. Accordingly, a procedure should be established that allows all board members to give the evaluation committee their opinions on setting evaluation criteria and their own evaluation judgments. Many boards have their members fill out a form that grades the CEO's performance in several areas of hospital activity. This cumulative grading can help the evaluation committee to determine the overall opinion of the members of the governing body and their perception of the CEO.

The most common period for which the CEO should be evaluated is the fiscal year of the institution. However, the calendar year or some other period may also be used, as long as it is an agreed-upon time that is suitable to all concerned.

In order to be as fair and impartial as possible, the evaluation should take place soon after the end of the time period agreed on. It is not desirable to wait for six months after the period has ended to do the evaluation. Some delay may be unavoidable or even necessary under certain circumstances, but this should be kept to a minimum. The time of evaluation should be clearly set forth in the written document, with a deadline for completion and a report to the full board on the results of the evaluation.

The findings of the evaluation committee should be in writing and, in addition to going to the full board, should be submitted to the CEO for any comment, with a written acknowledgment from the CEO. Only through this type of free and open communication between the board and the CEO will the evaluation be the effective process that it should be.

Evaluation needs to be an ongoing process. There is nothing wrong with looking at a CEO's performance in a given area on a quarterly or semiannual basis or some other interim time period. However, there should be a full understanding that the committee may desire or will undertake a critique of a particular matter or matters on an interim basis. An example of this might be a goal to reduce the hospital's uncollectible accounts by 5 percent within 12 months. The evaluation of this could well be on a quarterly or even monthly basis, so that the committee has an idea of just how this is going before the end of the 12-month period. Any number of matters lend themselves to an interim evaluation before the end of the period involved. If these areas can be agreed on by all of the parties, then the evaluation committee is that much ahead on its work.

Where such goal setting is used, it is often possible to assess the partial accomplishment of a task and not just give a rating based on full accomplishment or nothing. In the example just given, suppose the CEO has been able to reduce uncollectible accounts by 3.5 percent. Shouldn't there be some acknowledgment that this was accomplished, tempered by the fact that the agreed-upon goal was not accomplished? There could well be some mitigating circumstances that prohibited the full accomplishment of the goal.

It is essential that the evaluation process cover every aspect of the CEO's employment, from the day-to-day routine matters in the hospital to the most complex technological decision that may have to be made. No area in which the CEO functions should be overlooked or omitted. The committee has the prerogative to give weight and priority to the various areas on which it evaluates CEO performance, but the evaluation needs to look at the totality of the CEO's employment. Some CEOs will be stronger in some areas of employment than in others; they may have had more experience in one field of health care than another. Therefore, the evaluation committee has an even greater challenge to try to identify these strengths and weaknesses so that they can be assessed and thereby evaluated in the light of the entire scope of the CEO's work.

In addition to providing the basis for new or revised goal-setting, the outcome of the CEO's evaluation can be a useful tool in employment negotiations with the CEO. Often it may be a determining factor in pay, length of employment, or economic incentives. It should not be just a forgotten document allowed to gather dust on the shelf!

Checklist—Determining the Procedure

***Instructions:** Rate the following statements in relation to your hospital and governing board. Rank each statement from **5** (strongly agree) to **1** (strongly disagree) or answer **yes** or **no**.*

1.	The board has adopted a written policy dealing with CEO evaluation.	____Yes			____No	
2.	A committee of the board is appointed to evaluate the CEO's performance.	____Yes			____No	
3.	I think this committee is the right size to do this work.	5	4	3	2	1
4.	The committee seeks input from the entire board for the evaluation.	5	4	3	2	1
5.	A well-defined period of time is established for which the CEO will be evaluated.	5	4	3	2	1
6.	The committee makes a complete report to the board of its findings.	5	4	3	2	1
7.	In some instances the CEO is evaluated on an interim basis.	5	4	3	2	1
8.	I am satisfied that the evaluation process covers all aspects of the CEO's duties and responsibilities.	5	4	3	2	1
9.	The results of the evaluation are used in negotiations with the CEO regarding status of employment.	5	4	3	2	1
10.	The results of the evaluation are used in setting new goals for constructive change and improvement of performance.	5	4	3	2	1

Subjective and Objective Evaluation

By the very nature of the process, subjective as well as objective criteria will be part of the evaluation of the CEO. Both are important, but to ensure a fair evaluation, as much objectivity as possible is needed.

To help in distinguishing the two, here are some questions of opinion that fall in the subjective category: How well is the CEO liked in the community? Does the CEO have a good public relations image in the community? Is the CEO well respected by fellow health care professionals? Does the CEO get along well with the medical staff? Is the CEO visible in the institution? These types of questions are important to ask in the evaluation, but they are mainly the opinions of individuals and cannot be measured with precision.

Now consider some objective criteria that are easily quantifiable and therefore can be measured: Did the hospital operate within the budget? Did the building of the new wing proceed on the adopted schedule? Has contact been made and have plans been completed for networking with the neighboring hospital? Have the physicians been recruited that were needed for the expanded services the hospital wants to offer? What has been the turnover of employees by department for the past 12 months?

Subjective opinions must be expressed, including the important area of employees' opinions about the hospital and their work. One way to try to determine the mind-set of employees is through an attitude survey. (See the section Employee Relations on page 73 for more on this topic.) The evaluation committee must then consider the validity of these and other subjective opinions and must determine the proper weight to give them.

Mutual agreement is necessary in setting measurable, objective goals for the CEO. Otherwise, a board might hold the CEO solely responsible for a particular outcome even though other factors might affect the end result. Suppose, for example, the board charges the CEO with the responsibility to see that a much needed additional medical service is added at the institution. Any number of factors could affect the result, from the certificate-of-need process to specialized input from the medical staff, and it would not be fair to evaluate the CEO as if he or she were the only one responsible for the accomplishment of this goal. By a full and open discussion between both parties of the extent to which the

CEO can be held accountable, an agreement can be reached on which a fair evaluation of the CEO can be undertaken.

Goal statements that include objective means of evaluation should be put in writing and shared with all concerned, including the full board of the hospital. Doing this reduces the chance for misunderstanding and establishes an atmosphere of openness and trust, which is vital to the successful outcome of the process.

Checklist—Subjective and Objective Evaluation

Instructions: *Rate the following statements in relation to your hospital and governing board. Rank each statement from* ***5*** *(strongly agree) to* ***1*** *(strongly disagree).*

1. Objective, measurable goals are part of the CEO's evaluation.	5	4	3	2	1
2. I believe that the effort is made to handle the subjective areas of evaluation fairly and responsibly.	5	4	3	2	1
3. The evaluation process takes into consideration opinions from the community as well as from the institution.	5	4	3	2	1
4. I believe that the evaluation is fair and impartial.	5	4	3	2	1
5. Objective evaluation criteria are put in writing and shared with the full board.	5	4	3	2	1

The CEO's Role in Planning

Planning is essential to any health care institution, and therefore the CEO's role in planning is an important area of evaluation. This role encompasses both the CEO's contribution to the planning process and, of course, the CEO's effectiveness in carrying out those portions of the plans that are within the scope of his or her responsibility.

Mission Statement

Planning begins with the mission statement of the hospital, which should set forth clearly and succinctly just what the board expects in the way of health care delivery from the institution it governs. It is essential that the role of the CEO be in harmony with and supportive of these expectations, and for the CEO to be in agreement with this document. Adopting a mission statement should not be undertaken without input from the CEO and the executive staff of the hospital.

A clear understanding by the board and the CEO is necessary regarding those aspects of the mission statement that are within the CEO's area of responsibility, although this information may not be specified in the mission statement itself. These responsibilities, as well as information on the necessary time for accomplishment and the financial resources available, are usually specified in detail in other documents such as goals and objectives or an action plan for the CEO.

Checklist—Mission Statement

Instructions: *Rate the following statements in accordance with the facts of your hospital and governing board. Rank each statement from* ***5*** *(strongly agree) to* ***1*** *(strongly disagree).*

Statement					
1. The CEO has input in the preparation of the mission statement.	5	4	3	2	1
2. The board and the CEO agree on those aspects of the mission statement that are within the CEO's area of responsibility.	5	4	3	2	1
3. The mission statement is used as a basis for setting objectives in the evaluation of the CEO.	5	4	3	2	1

Long-Range/Strategic Plan

Often the CEO is the moving factor in the long-range or strategic planning process, whether it is done in-house or with some outside assistance.

The CEO, by the nature of his or her responsibility in the health care arena, should be the single individual in the hospital most knowledgeable about today's health care environment and the dynamics of change. This expertise is a necessary ingredient for the successful planning process, despite differences in individual leadership style. One CEO might prefer to comment and offer suggestions as plans are discussed; another might prefer to take a leadership position in putting forth ideas or thoughts concerning the present or future direction of the institution. Whatever the style, how effectively the CEO contributes to the planning process is an area for CEO evaluation.

The long-range plan should be regularly reviewed by the board or a board committee to make sure that the planning process is on target regarding the projects and time frames set forth. Because the CEO plays the single most important role in this regular review, this is also an opportune time to review the work of the CEO in implementing the hospital's plans.

Checklist—Long-Range/Strategic Plan

Instructions: *Rate the following statements in relation to your hospital and governing board. Rank each answer from* **5** *(strongly agree) to* **1** *(strongly disagree).*

1. The CEO plays a major role in the long-range or strategic planning process.	5	4	3	2	1
2. There is good understanding between the CEO and the board as to projects to be achieved under the long-range or strategic plan.	5	4	3	2	1

Specific Goals and Objectives

Once the plans of the hospital are established, specific goals and objectives need to be set to implement the plans. The role of the CEO in determining and carrying out these goals and objectives is of utmost importance and should be a high priority item in the evaluation process. Here again, it is important to have agreement between the board and the CEO on the goals and on the specific objectives that should be met in reaching the goals.

For example, consider the common practice of acquiring a parcel of real estate needed for the hospital's expansion. The CEO might be given a broad assignment to try to find out the purchase price of the real estate. In carrying out this assignment, the CEO might consider three courses of action: getting an appraisal of the property, contacting the owner directly to see if there was a price set on the property, or arranging to have someone anonymously inquire about the acquisition.

In this example, the board could avoid any misunderstanding by giving the CEO some specific guidelines, for example, saying to the CEO, "...so let's authorize an appraisal of the property not to exceed $450; after we receive the appraisal, we'll discuss the best method of approaching the owner." Wherever possible, it is best to specify what is expected of the CEO so that there is less chance for misunderstanding by all concerned. This does not mean that the CEO is so restricted in carrying out a task that all opportunity for initiative or innovation is taken away. That situation would be very counterproductive and would lead to destroying the leadership that is so necessary from the CEO.

Setting any goal or objective should include some kind of a time frame in which it is to be completed. To simply state a goal or objective that is not to be attained by any agreed-upon time is almost meaningless. The CEO or whoever is responsible for completion of such an undertaking must agree that the time set forth is realistic for attaining the objective.

Those specific goals and objectives that are within the scope of the CEO's responsibility may be further documented as an action or work plan, which becomes one basis for evaluation of the CEO's performance. Any work plan must clearly define what is expected of the CEO or the executive staff and must also address any areas of uncertainty. If goals and objectives are stated in specific, measurable terms whenever possible, the evaluation process will be more effective and will be fair to all concerned.

Checklist—Specific Goals and Objectives

Instructions: *Rate the following statements in relation to your hospital and governing board. Rank each answer from* **5** *(strongly agree) to* **1** *(strongly disagree).*

1. The board sets forth specific goals and objectives in accordance with the planning of the institution.	5	4	3	2	1
2. The board identifies those goals and objectives on which the CEO's performance will be evaluated.	5	4	3	2	1
3. The goals and objectives set forth are agreed upon by all concerned with the evaluation process.	5	4	3	2	1
4. Any specific task on which the CEO is to be evaluated clearly defines the role of the CEO in carrying it out.	5	4	3	2	1
5. Goals and objectives on which the CEO is to be evaluated have a realistic time frame in which to be accomplished.	5	4	3	2	1
6. Whenever possible, goals and objectives are set in such a manner that their accomplishment can be measured.	5	4	3	2	1

Day-to-Day Functions of the CEO

Most governing boards fully realize the role they play as a policy-making body rather than a body involved in the day-to-day operations of the institution. Although the board is not involved in the daily activities of the CEO, it *is* concerned about the leadership ability of the CEO in this arena because an organization that runs smoothly is most desirable for the effective handling of the hospital's affairs.

Leadership Ability

Different CEOs have different styles of leadership, and there is no way to set forth a model of administration. Nor should the board attempt to impose on the CEO some particular brand of leadership that it favors. However, boards are interested in some general areas of leadership, and these areas are important in the evaluation process.

- The governing body wants to see an efficiently run hospital that maintains a close working relationship between management and employees. To this extent management needs to have an open-door policy so that morale is good and employees know there is a way to pursue any grievance they may have. An administration that shuts itself off from its employees often will find itself in an adversarial role in employer-employee relations.
- Management needs to be visible in the institution on a regular basis to its employees. Tom Peters, author of *In*

Search of Excellence, talks about the successful CEO and "management by wandering around (MBWA)"! His point is the necessity for visibility to employees, thereby indicating a caring concern on the part of management.

- The CEO must have an excellent working team at the top level of management. Accordingly, the board needs to be assured that the necessary management personnel is present to carry out the executive functions that are so essential to a well-run organization.
- The board will be concerned by any organizational structure that seems top-heavy in administration or executive personnel and will often be critical of a CEO who so structures the executive staff. A CEO may avoid this reaction by keeping the board informed whenever top-level executives are hired and by setting forth the reasoning for this action.
- The board is always interested in the organizational structure of the hospital and just how various executive management responsibilities are delegated by the CEO to subordinates. This information needs to be shared with the board, and the rationale for such decisions could be an area of evaluation.
- The governing body likes to see a functional organization that is structured to produce the maximum efficiency without the appearance of excess personnel. Although it is sometimes difficult to achieve just the proper balance in this area, a CEO should always be aware of these constraints and should try for the proper balance in executive management and in the work load that is placed on certain positions.
- The board becomes concerned by what members perceive to be crisis management. This term describes an atmosphere of decision making under crisis conditions almost all of the time. There is no argument that there are crises in health care, and some hospitals will face a crisis at any given time, but the governing board should not accept the premise that crisis is a day-to-day way of life at its health care institution. The handling of a true crisis, however, is often used in the evaluation process.

Checklist—Leadership Ability

Instructions: *Rate the following statements in relation to your hospital and governing board. Rank each answer from* **5** *(strongly agree) to* **1** *(strongly disagree).*

1. The organizational structure of the hospital provides for an efficient, smooth-running management team.	5	4	3	2	1
2. The CEO and management staff are accessible to those employees who wish to see them.	5	4	3	2	1
4. A good working relationship exists among top-level management personnel.	5	4	3	2	1
5. The management of the hospital is handled in an orderly manner and is not crisis-oriented.	5	4	3	2	1

Employee Relations

The morale of employees is an important factor in the delivery of health care. Good employee morale can overcome many deficiencies that may exist in an institution, and, conversely, poor employee morale can detract from the finest medical technology.

Dozens of media accounts have described events like work stoppages, massive use of sick days, strikes, and so forth, that all indicate a morale problem in an institution. In today's competitive environment, the perceived attitude of employees may have a significant influence on where a prospective patient decides to seek medical care.

Not only does morale influence the public's opinion of the hospital and its quality of care, it also has a direct impact on the efficiency of operations. Poor or low morale can increase the cost of health care delivery and can have a dramatic effect on the bottom line of operations. Sloppiness in housekeeping, for example, by an employee who is just trying to pass the time as effortlessly as possible, can result in waste of materials and a job half done that has to be repeated. Good morale by workers who really set out to do a job in the best possible manner can cause a hospital to achieve maximum efficiency of operations and therefore produce the proper margin for its fiscal activity.

Poor employee morale also influences a physician's perception of the hospital and can play a major role in the determination of just where a patient might be placed for medical treatment. This matter, if it becomes a subject of general conversation in the community, can have a direct effect on the admittance pattern of the institution.

Some hospitals use an attitude survey to determine employees' feelings about their work. Although it is not completely effective in making known the exact feelings of employees, it is a fairly accurate measure of morale when administered properly by a professional in this field. It is probably the best method of determining employee morale that is available to management and that is not offensive to employees.

A number of factors need to be considered, however, in assessing the results of an attitude survey.

- An attitude survey can be affected by the timeliness of its undertaking; a survey taken immediately following some large layoff of employees or the closing of a wing might greatly affect the results and tend to give a much more adverse picture than actually exists.

- Most attitude surveys are completed anonymously, and this in itself may contribute to a distortion of true feelings under certain circumstances.
- When a hospital is dealing with a third party in a collective bargaining situation, an attitude survey may prove of very little, if any, benefit. However, some attitude surveys in a collective bargaining situation are invaluable in allowing a free expression of feelings among employees. The presence of a collective bargaining situation is something that should be kept in mind whenever an attitude survey is undertaken.

Looking at department turnover of personnel is another way to try to determine job satisfaction. Usually, a glaring disparity between one department and others is a red flag to indicate a possibility of a morale problem within the department with the high turnover. However, to use the rate of turnover as a sole means of determining employee morale could be misleading; this information should be used only in conjunction with more detailed studies. Needless to say, the replacement of personnel is a costly procedure that could account for a more expensive operation of a department than would be normally acceptable.

Checklist—Employee Relations

Instructions: *Rate the following statements in relation to your hospital and governing board. Rank each answer from* **5** *(strongly agree) to* **1** *(strongly disagree) or answer* **yes** *or* **no**.

1. Good employee morale exists in the hospital.	5 4 3 2 1
2. An employee attitude survey has been conducted by the hospital within the past three years.	____Yes ____No
3. A significant work stoppage or slowdown has not occurred during the past five years.	____Yes ____No
4. Employee turnover is at an acceptable level in all departments.	5 4 3 2 1
5. There are no excessive costs due to low levels of employee performance.	5 4 3 2 1

Board-Management Relations

It has been stated over and over again that governing boards have no place in the daily management of the institution. This is a sound axiom. Although boards may occasionally foray into the operational activities of the hospital, this should be minimal and a rare occurrence. Nothing undermines the leadership ability of a CEO more than having a board or individuals from the board continually interject themselves into the daily operations of the institution. This is truly a counterproductive activity that will in all probability lead to friction between the board and administration.

In matters of corporate leadership concerning both the board and executive management, what is expected of the governing board and what is expected of executive management should be clearly defined so that neither infringes on the other's area of responsibility. Boards may respond at any time when their advice is sought in this area of day-to-day management, and, likewise, management's advice is most appropriate in the policy-making area of governance, but each must clearly understand that advice is not to be confused with final responsibility. The successful running of a health care institution is based on this understanding. Just how top management deals with this relationship is going to be of utmost importance to those responsible for the evaluation of the CEO.

Checklist—Board-Management Relations

Instructions: *Rate the following statements in relation to your hospital and governing board. Rank each answer from* **5** *(strongly agree) to* **1** *(strongly disagree).*

1. The CEO is comfortable in asking opinions of the board that might relate to management of the hospital.	5	4	3	2	1
2. Neither the board nor any individual board member becomes routinely involved in the day-to-day operation of the hospital.	5	4	3	2	1

Role in the Community

In most instances the CEO is seen as the single person most representative of the hospital. Therefore, at all times the CEO should remember that this public perception follows wherever he or she goes. The CEO is expected to be the hospital's representative in all areas of community life, from everyday civic activities to the most complex negotiations with a government authority. The visibility of the CEO is of vital importance to the institution and therefore of great concern to the governing board in its evaluation of performance. No other person has the unique position that the CEO does in affecting the public's opinion of the hospital.

Rightly or wrongly, the hospital is often judged on the behavior of the CEO in the community and the impression he or she gives. Governing boards must be aware of this impression and must be able to relate it to the overall well-being of the institution.

It is important here to be able to separate the wheat from the chaff. The board cannot rely solely on what the public may think of the CEO nor can it ignore this entirely; it has to balance this opinion along with all the other opinions it gets, in order to evaluate the CEO accurately and fairly.

Checklist—Role in the Community

Instructions: *Rate the following statements in relation to your hospital and governing board. Rank each answer from **5** (strongly agree) to **1** (strongly disagree).*

1. The CEO is active in the community in various civic affairs.	5	4	3	2	1
2. The CEO is visible in the community and is recognized as the representative of the hospital.	5	4	3	2	1
3. The CEO is a good public relations emissary in the community the hospital serves.	5	4	3	2	1

Medical Staff-Management Relations

Perhaps the most challenging day-to-day function of the CEO is handling the relationship between this position and the medical staff of the institution. If information is ever compiled on the reasons for CEOs leaving a hospital, whether voluntary or forced, my opinion is that the medical staff-CEO relationship would rank very high, if not at the top.

In most instances the first contact that a new member of the medical staff has with the hospital is at the CEO level. Here first impressions are important and can often set the course for behavior patterns by the new physician.

Because so much of the relationship is often dependent on individual personalities, it is difficult to set forth any guidelines for, or characteristics of, good medical staff-CEO relations. What works in one hospital may not work in another; a success story in one situation may become a disaster when tried under different circumstances. Nevertheless, this relationship requires evaluation and is most important in assessing the performance of the CEO.

A hospital may exist without good medical staff-CEO relations, but it will exist in an atmosphere that is not conducive to attaining the high quality of care that should be the goal of any health care institution. In addition, a CEO that has to function in this atmosphere may feel so threatened as to be ineffective in other areas of activity that are not even related to medical staff concerns.

In the dynamics of today's health care delivery system, with increased competition between doctors and hospitals and with joint ventures becoming an accepted practice, the medical staff-CEO relationship is of greater importance than ever before. Indeed, this relationship is of such importance that it will in all probability be reflected either as an asset or a liability in all other areas of the hospital; it is therefore quite understandable why a governing board would give it such a high priority in the evaluation process.

Checklist—Medical Staff-Management Relations

Instructions: *Rate the following statements in relation to your hospital and governing board. Rank each answer from* **5** *(strongly agree) to* **1** *(strongly disagree).*

1. A good relationship exists between the CEO and the medical staff.	5	4	3	2	1
2. Harmful competitive situations do not exist between the hospital and the medical staff.	5	4	3	2	1

Contracts for the CEO

Until recent years, contracts for the CEO have been a rather rare item. With the complexity of the health care environment, they have become more and more a standard way of delineating the employment agreement between the hospital and its CEO. As the health care delivery system comes under greater pressures and as competition increases among all the segments of the industry, contracts are expected to become even more popular in the employment relationship. Because CEOs are sometimes forced into adversarial relations with the medical staff, third-party payers, business entities, employees, and in even rare instances the governing body, they are increasingly aware of the need for some kind of protection from the emotionalism that may accompany these relationships.

The governing body as a whole needs to be aware of any contract that is used in the employment of the CEO and should at least be informed of the major provisions of such a contract. However, in negotiating a contract with the CEO, only a small group should be involved. Usually the executive committee or some such small committee of the board will be delegated the authority to do the preliminary negotiating, with the full board being responsible for the final approval.

Contracts of employment should be confidential and so regarded by all of the parties concerned. Some details of the contract may have to be made public under certain circumstances, but such disclosure should be kept to a minimum. Because contracts are legally binding, they must be reviewed and approved by qualified legal counsel. It is not uncommon for the prospective CEO to ask for legal review by his or her own attorney as well.

Contracts between the two parties must be bilateral. The contract that is written totally in the interest of the institution and does not fairly represent the interest of the CEO will be of no benefit when it comes under close scrutiny. Likewise, a contract that is nothing more than a separation agreement between the hospital and the CEO should be labeled as that and not as a contract of employment. I do not mean to minimize the importance of separation and the place it has in the contract, but if the contract deals only with separation, in my opinion it is not an employment contract but a separation contract and should be viewed in that light.

Governing boards sometimes have a difficult time understanding their responsibility when a CEO is discharged. They may be under the impression that they had a clear right to do what they did, only to find out that the contract under which the CEO was working specified something different. Fairness to both parties is a complex thing to arrive at and an even more difficult thing to put down in writing, but it must be done or there may be dire consequences when the enforcement of a contract becomes necessary.

A governing body may wish some outside help when faced with preparing a contract. It has been often said in law and the fringe areas of it that a poorly written contract is a source of great income for attorneys! Do not be misled, however, into thinking that the best written contract possible will guarantee freedom from litigation at some time. The goal of all concerned should be a contract that is rarely invoked but when necessary will resolve any differences that may arise between the CEO and the hospital.

Checklist—Contracts for the CEO

Instructions: *Rate the following statements in relation to your hospital and governing board (only for those institutions with contracts). Rank each statement from* **5** *(strongly agree) to* **1** *(strongly disagree) or answer* ***yes*** *or* ***no****.*

1.	As a board member I am familiar with the contract with the CEO.	5	4	3	2	1
2.	A relatively small committee of the board handles negotiations with the CEO.	5	4	3	2	1
3.	All negotiations between the CEO and the institution require final approval by the full governing board.	5	4	3	2	1
4.	The contract has been reviewed by an attorney.	____Yes			____No	
5.	I believe the contract is fair to both parties.	5	4	3	2	1
6.	In my opinion, the contract covers all the areas of employment that are pertinent to the position of CEO.	5	4	3	2	1
7.	The contract is reviewed on a regular basis with the CEO.	5	4	3	2	1

Incentive Compensation for Executive Management

Economic incentives have been around for a long time, but usually more in the business and industrial area of our economy than in health care. Although late in arriving in the health care field, they are increasing at a rapid rate, fueled by the corporate restructuring that has taken place recently. The possible advantages of an incentive plan to the hospital are many, including improved employee morale, productivity, executive retention, and financial savings. Little wonder that incentives for the executive management of a health care institution are of increasing popularity!

There are many ways of providing incentives. Some hospitals give incentives at various levels of employment as a means of encouraging those seeking promotion within the organization. These can be such things as vacation days, use of an automobile, amount of life insurance, club membership fees, dependent travel, and use of recreational facilities. This section, however, deals only with incentive compensation.

Incentive compensation is designed to recognize and reward exceptional performance of an individual by means of compensation above the regular salary. It should not be confused with merit pay, which is usually administered to employees by management personnel. The possibility of incentive compensation should never be used as a substitute for fair pay or the standard salary that is due an individual for fulfilling the expected duties of employment.

An incentive compensation plan is an objective method of evaluating and rewarding performance. Although subjectivity may be a part of other kinds of evaluation, it has no place in evaluation for incentive compensation. This plan must be linked to a performance evaluation and must use definable and agreed-upon goals.

When these goals are met or surpassed, the hospital usually achieves a considerable financial saving that far offsets the cost of the plan.

Incentive compensation is normally restricted to the top echelon of executive management. In most instances the incentive compensation plan for the CEO is administered by a rather small, select committee of the board. For others in executive management positions, it is usually administered by the CEO under a plan approved by the governing body or a committee thereof. If incentive plans are extended to the department level, a further delegation of responsibility is needed for their administration.

An incentive compensation plan can provide many benefits to all concerned, but it is a complex undertaking that requires careful study. An institution that is considering the use of incentive compensation should probably seek some professional help in adopting such a plan.

Checklist—Incentive Compensation for Executive Management

Instructions: *If your hospital has an incentive pay plan, rate the following statements in relation to your hospital and governing board. Rank each statement from* **5** *(strongly agree) to* **1** *(strongly disagree).*

Statement					
1. The incentive pay plan is administered in an objective manner.	5	4	3	2	1
2. The board approves the incentive pay plan for executive management.	5	4	3	2	1
3. The board is informed of the performance of those individuals receiving incentive compensation.	5	4	3	2	1
4. The board has input into the goals set for executive management under the incentive plan.	5	4	3	2	1
5. I think the incentive compensation plan is accomplishing its purpose and benefiting the institution.	5	4	3	2	1

About the Author

Richard P. Moses is a trustee of Tuomey Hospital, Sumter, South Carolina, a member of the Board of Trustees of the American Hospital Association, and a former consulting director for the AHA Program for Hospital Governing Boards.

Long active in the health care field, he is a former chairman of the South Carolina Hospital Association and of the Policy Advisory Committee of the Joint Commission on Accreditation of Hospitals. He also served on the National Commission on Nursing and is an honorary fellow of the American College of Healthcare Executives.

Mr. Moses is a frequent speaker on health care governance and is currently a consultant to the Board Effectiveness Evaluation Program of the Illinois Hospital Association, a project encompassing on-site consultations at 22 Illinois hospitals.

He is a graduate of the University of North Carolina and a former mayor of Sumter, South Carolina, where he is vice-president of a real estate company.